ESSENTIAL GUIDE TO MYCOSIS FUNGOLDES

Comprehensive Insights and Treatment Strategies for Practitioners and Patients

DR. CASEY LOREN

DISCLAIMER

This book's content is only meant to be used for general informative purposes. Although the author has taken great care to ensure the content is accurate and thorough, no warranties or assurances on the information's accuracy, correctness, or reliability are provided. It is recommended that readers employ their own judgment and discretion when applying any material found in this book to their particular situation.

The information in this book is not intended to replace professional advice, nor is the author an expert in any of the subjects covered. It is recommended that readers consult with experienced professionals regarding any particular issues or concerns.

Any name that may be mentioned or referred in this book does not imply endorsement, recommendation, or relationship on the part of the author with any person, entity, good, website, or association. These references are made only for informational purposes and are not meant to be taken as recommendations or endorsements.

The information contained in this book may cause readers to suffer loss or damage, for which the author disclaims all obligation and accountability. The only people accountable for the decisions and actions taken by readers using the information presented are themselves.

Any names, characters, companies, locations, activities, occasions, and incidents referenced in this book are either made up or the result of the author's imagination. Any likeness to real people, living or dead, or to real things is entirely coincidental.

This book's content may change at any time, without prior notice, according to the author. The onus is on the reader to verify whether there have been any updates or revisions.

The reader accepts the conditions of this disclaimer by reading this book. Please do not

read this book or use its contents if you do not
agree to these terms.

CHAPTER 1

OVERVIEW OF MYCOSIS FUNGOIDES

Explanation and Synopsis of Mycosis Fungoides

A rare kind of non-Hodgkin lymphoma that mostly affects the skin is called mycosis fungoides. It is a member of a class of illnesses known as cutaneous T-cell lymphomas, which are distinguished by T-cells proliferating abnormally in the skin. Mycosis fungoides, despite its name, is caused by aberrant T-cell activity rather than a fungus. It can be difficult to diagnose because the disorder progresses slowly over many years and frequently appears first as a rash or patchy region of discolored skin that may resemble other skin conditions.

Historical Context and Findings

Mycosis fungoides was initially documented in 1806 by French dermatologist Jean-Louis-Marc Alibert, which puts its history in the early 1800s. The condition was originally known as "granuloma fongueux de la peau," or "fungoid granuloma of the skin," but English dermatologist Malcolm Morris renamed it mycosis fungoides in 1892. Since then, substantial progress has been made in our knowledge of the pathophysiology, diagnosis, and management of the illness.

Prevalence and Epidemiology

Mycosis fungoides is regarded as an uncommon illness, making around 0.5–1% of all lymphomas. Adults between the ages of 40 and 60 are usually affected, with men experiencing the condition slightly more frequently than women. Geographically, the prevalence varies; higher rates have been reported in some areas. Although the precise etiology of mycosis fungoides is still unknown, scientists think immune system, environmental, and genetic variables may be involved in the disease's development.

Causes and Risk Elements

Although the precise cause of mycosis fungoides is uncertain, several factors may play a role in its emergence. These include immune system failure, viral infections, exposure to certain chemicals or environmental pollutants, and genetic predisposition. Mycosis fungoides may be more common in people with a family history of lymphomas or autoimmune disorders.

Symptoms and Clinical Manifestations

Typically, mycosis fungoides manifests as skin-related symptoms, which can differ greatly in intensity and appearance. Red, scaly patches or plaques that resemble psoriasis or eczema are examples of early-stage symptoms. As the condition worsens, symptoms like ulceration, pruritus, thicker, elevated lesions (tumors), and enlarged lymph nodes may appear. When mycosis fungoides reaches an advanced stage, it can affect internal organs and cause systemic symptoms like fever, exhaustion, and weight loss.

Medical Procedures

A combination of clinical assessment, skin samples, imaging techniques, and laboratory testing is frequently needed to diagnose mycosis fungoides. A comprehensive physical examination can be conducted by dermatologists and oncologists to evaluate skin lesions and lymph nodes. A skin sample is necessary to confirm the diagnosis because aberrant T-cell infiltration in the skin layers is shown by histological investigation. Tests such as blood work, imaging (CT scans, for example), and molecular studies might be performed in addition to the above to determine the severity of the disease and rule out other disorders.

Scenario and Outlook

Determining the degree of skin involvement, lymph node enlargement, and possible organ involvement are important steps in the staging of mycosis fungoides. The TNMB classification, which classifies the disease based on tumor size, node involvement, metastasis, and blood involvement, is the staging approach that is most frequently employed. The prognosis differs significantly depending on the stage of the disease at diagnosis; in general, early-stage disease has a better prognosis than advanced-stage disease. To track the course of the disease and the effectiveness of treatment, routine follow-up evaluations, and monitoring are essential.

Medical Strategies

The goals of mycosis fungoides treatment are to manage the disease's course, reduce symptoms, and enhance quality of life. The stage of the disease, the level of involvement, and the unique characteristics of each patient all influence the therapy option. Topical drugs (corticosteroids, retinoids), phototherapy (UV light therapy), systemic treatments (chemotherapy, targeted therapies, immunotherapy), and radiation therapy are examples of common therapeutic techniques. For refractory or severe disease, clinical trials and experimental medicines may be taken into consideration in some situations.

Recent Studies and Advancements

The goals of current mycosis fungoides research are to better understand the disease's causes, find new therapy targets, and enhance patient outcomes. Technological developments in immunotherapy, targeted medicines, and molecular profiling offer hope for more individualized and efficient treatment plans. Clinical trials assessing novel medications, combination treatments, and immunomodulatory agents are actively influencing the management of mycosis fungoides.

To sum up, mycosis fungoides is a complicated lymphoproliferative illness with unique pathological and clinical characteristics. Though uncommon, the condition can have a major impact on patients' lives, requiring thorough knowledge, prompt diagnosis, and customized treatment plans. Research endeavors and partnerships must persist to augment our understanding, improve diagnostic techniques, and progress treatment alternatives for those afflicted with mycosis fungoides.

CHAPTER 2

THE PATHOPHYSIOLOGY OF FUNGAL MYCOSIS

Mycosis Fungoides Pathogenesis

Determining the origin, course, and possible targets for the treatment of Mycosis Fungoides (MF), a kind of cutaneous T-cell lymphoma, requires an understanding of its pathophysiology. Let's explore every facet of MF etiology in detail.

Anatomy and Function of the Skin

The skin is the biggest organ in the body, controlling temperature and fluid balance as well as acting as a barrier against external toxins. It is made up of several layers, such as the dermis, epidermis, and subcutaneous tissue, each of which has a different purpose in immunity and skin function.

Immunological Underpinnings of Fungoides Mycosis

Abnormal immunological responses, especially those involving T cells, are a hallmark of multiple sclerosis. When normal immune surveillance mechanisms are dysregulated, cancerous T-cells infiltrate the skin and eventually form tumors.

T-Cells' Function in the Pathogenesis of Disease

Malignant T-cells, usually belonging to the CD4+ class, are essential to the pathophysiology of MF. These cells have changed routes for activation, proliferation, and survival; as a result, they accumulate in the skin and produce distinctive tumors and plaques.

Environmental and Genetic Factors

Although the precise origin of MF is yet unknown, environmental factors and genetic predisposition probably play a role. People may be predisposed to MF by genetic changes that impact T-cell receptor signaling, cell cycle regulation, and immune response pathways. Viral infections and ultraviolet (UV) radiation are two other environmental triggers that have been linked to the development of disease.

Inflammatory Routes Activated

One of the main characteristics of MF is chronic inflammation, and inflammatory mediators, chemokines, and cytokines all have a major part in how the illness progresses. Tumour growth is further promoted by dysregulated inflammatory pathways, which also play a role in T-cell activation, recruitment, and tissue destruction.

Chemokines and Cytokines in the Progression of Disease

In MF, there is dysregulation of several cytokines and chemokines that affect angiogenesis, immune cell recruitment, and tumor microenvironment modification. Examples that contribute to the inflammatory milieu and disease development are IL-2, IL-10, IL-12, TNF-alpha, CCL17, and CCL22, among others.

Mechanisms of Immune Evasion

To avoid being recognized and eliminated by the immune system, malignant T-cells in MF use immune evasion techniques. These methods could involve the production of immunosuppressive factors, the downregulation of antigen-presenting molecules, and the suppression of T-cell activation and function.

Microbiome's Effect on Illness

There is growing evidence that the skin microbiota may play a part in the pathophysiology of MF. Changes in the microbial communities on the skin's surface can affect inflammation, the course of a disease, and local immunological responses. To fully understand the intricate relationships between the microbiota and MF, more investigation is required.

New Theories and Theories in Emergence

Novel insights into the pathophysiology of MF are still being uncovered by ongoing research, including:

- How epigenetic changes affect how genes are expressed and how cells function in MF.

- Potential targets for immunotherapy include immune evasion pathways and immune checkpoint dysregulation.

- Interactions that affect the course of the disease between stromal cells and malignant T-cells in the tumor microenvironment.

In conclusion, mycosis fungoides is a complicated illness with multiple etiology combining immunological, microbiological, environmental, and genetic components. Dysregulated inflammatory pathways, aberrant T-cell responses, immune evasion strategies, and interactions within the tumor microenvironment contribute to disease progression. Emerging research continues to expand our understanding of MF etiology and may lead to breakthrough treatment methods targeting important molecular and immunological pathways.

CHAPTER 3

CLINICAL PRESENTATION AND VARIANTS

Classic Presentations of Mycosis Fungoides

The most prevalent type of cutaneous T-cell lymphoma, known as mycosis fungoides, is predominantly characterized by skin involvement. Traditional presentations usually move through several phases:

1. **Patch Stage**: This first phase appears as erythematous (red), flat patches that may mimic psoriasis or eczema. The patches can be slightly irritating, but they are frequently asymptomatic.

2. **Plaque Stage**: The patches become thicker and eventually form plaques as the disease advances. These plaques have more noticeable erythema, are elevated, and may be scaly. They may have asymmetrical sizes and shapes.

3. **Tumour Stage**: Tumours or nodules may appear in later stages. These can develop ulcers and have an elevated, dome-shaped form. The tumors suggest a larger disease burden and deeper skin involvement.

Variants of Hypopigmented and Pigmented Skin

There are pigmentation differences in mycosis fungoides:

1. **Hypopigmented Variant**: This variant appears as lighter areas of skin and is more common in children and adults with darker complexion. It's possible to confuse these patches for vitiligo or other hypopigmentation conditions.

2. **Pigmented Variant**: This less frequent variation consists of darker, hyperpigmented spots or plaques. Since this variety resembles other hyperpigmented dermatoses, diagnosis can be more difficult.

Pagetoid and Folliculotropic Reticulosis Types

These variations differ in their histological and clinical characteristics:

1. **Folliculotropic Mycosis Fungoides**: This type of disease affects the hair follicles and frequently manifests as cysts, follicular papules, or acneiform lesions. It is frequently more treatment-resistant and may be connected to alopecia (hair loss).

2. **Pagetoid Reticulosis**: An uncommon kind that usually affects the limbs, with isolated or localized patches or plaques. It is characterized by the presence of abnormal lymphocytes in the epidermis and has a slow progression.

Sézary Syndrome: A Different Perspective

Different from mycosis fungoides, cutaneous T-cell lymphoma in an aggressive form is known as Sézary syndrome:

1. **Clinical Features**: It manifests as lymphadenopathy (enlarged lymph nodes), erythroderma (diffuse redness of the skin), and blood malignant T-cells (Sézary cells).

2. **Diagnostic Criteria**: The presence of Sézary cells in peripheral blood, histology, and clinical presentation are all necessary for the diagnosis. Molecular investigations and flow cytometry aid in the diagnosis confirmation.

Transdermal Involvement

In more advanced stages, mycosis fungoides can affect organs other than the skin:

1. **Nodes Lymphatic**: Frequently impacted, resulting in lymphadenopathy.

2. **Visceral Involvement**: Symptoms specific to the liver, spleen, and lungs may be present.

3. **Bone Marrow**: Involvement here can result in pancytopenia and is associated with a bad prognosis.

Age-Related and Paediatric Issues

How mycosis fungoides is presented and managed varies greatly with age:

1. **Paediatric Considerations**: Has a usually better prognosis and is more likely to present with hypopigmented lesions. Long-term therapeutic side effects must be taken into account by management.

2. **Geriatric Considerations**: Frequently manifests with more aggressive disease and at a later stage. The prognosis and choices for therapy are influenced by comorbidities and general health.

Difficulties with Differential Diagnosis

Mycosis fungoides resembles various dermatoses, making diagnosis difficult:

1. **Psoriasis/Eczema**: In its early stages, these common skin disorders might be mistaken for each other.

2. **Lichen Planus**: The plaque stage may mimic lichen planus; therefore, to make a precise diagnosis, immunohistochemical tests and biopsy are required.

3. **Drug Eruptions**: To distinguish between drug reactions that present similarly, a complete medication history and potential drug discontinuation may be necessary.

Emitting Parties and Converging Circumstances

Diagnosis can be complicated by certain illnesses that closely resemble mycosis fungoides.

1. **Parapsoriasis**: Long-term dermatoses akin to mycosis fungicides patch stage. Frequently, the differentiation is histological.

2. **Chronic Dermatitis**: Early mycosis fungoides can be mistaken for persistent dermatitis. Regular biopsies and careful clinical monitoring are necessary.

Clinical Scenarios and Case Studies

Thorough case studies offer useful information about the diagnosis and treatment of mycosis fungoides:

1. **Case Study 1**: This case study emphasizes the significance of biopsy in chronic dermatoses, with a middle-aged man presenting with persistent patches misdiagnosed as psoriasis for years.

2. **Case Study 2**: A young patient treated for vitiligo initially had hypopigmented patches; nevertheless, a subsequent diagnosis of mycosis

fungoides highlighted the importance of taking MF into account when making a differential diagnosis.

The "Essential Guide to Mycosis Fungoides" goes into great detail about the disease's many clinical manifestations and variations in Chapter 3. Accurate diagnosis and efficient treatment depend on an understanding of these various forms and the subtleties in their presentation. The significance of differentiating mycosis fungoides from related disorders using a thorough clinical assessment and suitable application of diagnostic instruments is also covered in this chapter.

CHAPTER 4

METHODS OF DIAGNOSIS

Doing a clinical examination and taking a history

Medical Assessment:

1. **Visual Inspection:** Extensive assessment of the whole skin surface to detect lesions, such as erythroderma, tumors, plaques, and patches, typical of Mycosis Fungoides (MF).

2. Using palpation, determine the depth, stiffness, and texture of skin lesions. Feel the lymph nodes for swelling.

3. **Documentation:** Standardised body maps and photos are used to record the progression and size of lesions.

Taking History:

1. **Symptom Onset and Duration:** Document the onset and development of skin lesions.

2. **Previous Treatments:** Record the outcomes of previous dermatological treatments.

3. **Family and Personal Medical History:** Mention any history of skin issues, autoimmune diseases, and other cancers.

4. **Systemic Symptoms:** Ask about fatigue, night sweats, pruritus, and weight loss.

Results of Dermoscopy in Mycosis Fungoides

Results from dermoscopy:

1. **Patch Stage:** Orange-yellowish patches, fine scales, and short, linear vessels (crown vessels).

2. **Plaque Stage:** Focus areas of crust/scale, linear vessels, and a background of yellow-orange.

3. Polymorphous arteries, ulcerations, and nodular features are indicative of the tumor stage.

4. **Utility of Dermoscopy:** Non-invasive, helps identify MF from other dermatoses and directs biopsy sites.

Methods for Skin Biopsy and Their Interpretation

Biopsy Methodologies:

1. **Punch Biopsy:** Often utilized, yields fully thick skin samples.

2. For deeper or larger lesions, use an incisional or excisional biopsy.

3. **Shave Biopsy:** May not be sufficient for deep infiltration, although occasionally used for superficial lesions.

Explanation:

1. **Histopathological Features:** Pautrier microabscesses, a band-like infiltrate in the dermis, and atypical lymphocytes in the epidermis (epidermotropism).

2. **Staging:** Depending on the degree and location of lymphocyte infiltration as well as the existence of large cell lymphoma transformation.

Markers for Immunohistochemistry

Standard Markers:

1. T-cell markers **CD3, CD4, and CD8:**, with MF usually exhibiting a CD4+ preponderance.

2. **CD30:** A marker indicating the transformation of big cells.

3. **CD7 and CD26:** frequently absent from MF cells, helping to distinguish them from benign circumstances.

4. Higher levels of the proliferation marker **Ki-67:** indicate an aggressive illness.

Diagnostics Molecular (PCR, FISH, etc.)

Polymerase Chain Reaction, or **PCR:

1. **TCR Gene Rearrangement:** Verifies malignancy by identifying clonal T-cell populations.

2. **Specificity and Sensitivity:** Excellent specificity, but necessitates supporting histology and clinical data.

In Situ Fluorescence Hybridization, or FISH:

1. **Chromosome Aberrations:** Defines particular genetic alterations linked to multiple sclerosis.

2. **Application:** Beneficial in situations where the immunophenotype or histology is unusual.

Imaging Research (MRI, PET-CT, CT)

Computerised Tomography (CT):

1. **Assessment:** Considers visceral and nodal involvement.

2. **Utility:** Helpful in tracking the course of diseases and staging them.

*Magnetic Resonance Imaging (MRI):

1. **Evaluation of Soft Tissue:** Excellent for determining skin and soft tissue involvement.

2. **Role:** Mostly restricted to particular indications requiring in-depth soft tissue resolution.

Electron Emission Tomography, or PET-CT:

1. **Metabolic Activity:** Identifies illness areas with metabolic activity.

2. **Application:** Relapse detection, therapy response assessment, and staging.

Serological and Blood Testing

Schedule Exams:

1. **Complete Blood Count (CBC):** Identifies cytopenias, which could point to involvement of the bone marrow.

2. **LDH (Lactate Dehydrogenase):** Increased levels are associated with a higher burden of disease.

Particular Examinations:

1. **Peripheral Blood Flow Cytometry:** Recognises cancerous T-cells (Sezary cells) in circulation.

2. **T-cell Clonality Assays** Verifies that clonal T-cell populations are present in blood.

Considerations for Lymph Node Biopsy

Significance:

1. **Clinical Enlarged Nodes:** Any nodes larger than 1.5 cm, especially if they are hard and not tender.

2. **Systemic Symptoms:** B symptoms (fever, sweats at night, and weight loss) are present.

Method:

1. **Excisional Biopsy:** Recommended for a thorough histological evaluation.

2. When excisional biopsy is not practical, consider a core needle biopsy as an alternative.

Explanation:

1. **Histological Patterns:** Complete effacement by malignant cells, paracortical enlargement, or dermatopathic lymphadenopathy.

2. **Immunophenotyping:** Assists in separating reactive conditions from MF.

Application of Cutting-Edge Technology

Generation-Next Sequencing (NGS):

1. **Genomic Profiling:** Identifies treatment targets and the mutations causing MF.

2. **Personalised Medicine:** Informs choices on targeted treatment.

Digital Pathology:

1. **Automated Image Analysis:** Improves the repeatability and precision of histopathology analyses.

2. **Telepathology:** Enables remote diagnoses and professional consultations.

Intellectual Property (IP):

1. **Pattern Recognition**: **Helps in lesion classification and early detection.

2. **Predictive Analytics:** makes predictions about treatment responses and outcomes by analyzing big datasets.

A thorough review of the diagnostic approaches for Mycosis Fungoides was given in this chapter, emphasizing the significance of combining cutting-edge molecular, histological, and clinical methods for precise diagnosis and staging. The importance of a comprehensive clinical examination, taking a thorough history, and using a range of diagnostic techniques—from dermoscopy to state-of-the-art molecular diagnostics—to guarantee an accurate diagnosis and successful treatment of mycosis fungoides are among the main lessons learned.

CHAPTER 5

PROGNOSTIC AND STAGING FACTORS

TNMB Categorization Scheme

Mycosis fungoides is a kind of cutaneous T-cell lymphoma that is evaluated and categorized using the TNMB classification system, a standardized staging technique. Tumour, Node, Metastasis, and Blood are the acronyms for this approach, and each one evaluates the disease's spread in a distinct area:

- **Tumour (T)**: Evaluates the degree of skin penetration.

- T1: Less than 10% of the skin's surface is covered with patches or plaques.

T2: Plaques or patches that cover ten percent or more of the skin's surface.

- T3: A single or more tumours (diameter ≥ 1 cm).

- T4: Erythema confluence encompassing 80% or more of the body's surface.

- **Node (N)**: Assesses lymph node involvement.

- N0: There are neither biopsy-negative nor palpably felt lymph nodes.

Palpable lymph nodes that are not histologically implicated (N1).

- N2: Palpable lymph nodes that do not fit the N3 criteria but are histologically involved.

- N3: Histologically affected lymph nodes exhibiting either whole or partial nodal architecture effacement.

The presence of extracutaneous involvement is indicated by the symbol **Metastasis (M)**.

M0: There is no visceral engagement.

- M1: Liver and lungs are examples of visceral involvement.

- **Blood (B)**: Determines whether the blood contains any cancerous T-cells.

- B0: Minimal involvement of blood.

- B1: Less than 5% of peripheral blood lymphocytes have blood tumors.

- B2: Elevated blood tumor load (more than 5% of peripheral blood cells).

Planning for staging and therapy requires a thorough and accurate assessment of the disease, which is made possible by the TNMB system.

Sentinel lymph node biopsy's function

A minimally invasive technique called sentinel lymph node biopsy (SLNB) is performed to assess if mycosis fungoides have progressed to the lymph nodes. The process entails the injection of radioactive material and/or dye in the vicinity of the tumor site to detect the initial lymph node (sentinel node) to drain the region. After surgery, this node is removed, and its cells are checked for malignancy.

- **SLNB Advantages**:

- Accurate Staging: By identifying microscopic metastases, aids in accurate staging.

- Treatment Planning: Affects choices about how much radiation, surgery, and systemic therapy are administered.

- Prognostic Data: Offers insightful prognostic data that help direct management and follow-up plans.

Treatment Planning's Crucial Role of Staging

It is important to stage mycosis fungoides for several reasons.

- **Guiding Treatment**: Different treatment modalities are needed depending on the stage of mycosis fungoides. Skin-directed therapy may be used to treat early-stage disease (Stage I–IIA), although systemic treatments are typically required for subsequent stages (Stage IIB–IV).

- **Predicting Outcomes**: The prognosis of the patient is predicted by staging. In general, the prognosis for early-stage disease is better than that of advanced stages.

- **Clinical Trials**: By ensuring suitable patient selection for clinical trials, staging contributes to the advancement of novel treatments.

Risk stratification and prognostic factors

The following variables affect the prognosis of mycosis fungoides:

- **Stage at Diagnosis**: The prognosis is better in earlier stages.

- **Histologic Subtype**: The prognosis may be worse for some subtypes, such as folliculotropic mycosis fungoides.

Large Cell Transformation: This suggests a more aggressive course of the illness and a less favorable prognosis.

Age and Sex: A worse prognosis is frequently linked to older age and male sex.

- **Level of Skin Involvement**: A disease that is more aggressive and advanced may have a significant skin involvement.

By combining these variables, risk stratification divides patients into several risk categories, directing the course of treatment and frequency of follow-up visits.

Genetic profiling and predictive biomarkers

Genetic profiling and biomarkers are two new tools in the management of mycosis fungoides:

- **Predictive Biomarkers**: Therapy response can be predicted by identifying particular biomarkers. One way to measure responsiveness to brentuximab vedotin is through CD30 expression.

- **Genetic Profiling**: Variations in genes that affect function, including mutations in TET2, DNMT3A, and RHOA, can reveal information about the etiology of a disease and suggest possible targets for treatment.

- **Personalised Medicine**: By customizing medicines according to each patient's unique genetic and molecular profile, these technologies allow for a more individualized approach that may lead to better results.

The Prognostic Effects of Age, Sex, and Race

Race, sex, and age all have a big influence on mycosis fungoides prognosis:

- **Age**: Older Patients typically have more advanced disease when they first arrive, and their prognosis is worse because of comorbidities and weaker therapeutic responses.

- **Sex**: Male patients typically have a poorer prognosis, which could be brought on by genetic or hormonal causes.

- **Race**: Due to genetic variations and unequal access to healthcare, some racial groups, such as African Americans, may exhibit more aggressive disease and poorer outcomes.

Suggestions for Extended-Term Monitoring

For patients with mycosis fungoides, long-term monitoring is essential:

- **Regular Monitoring**: To identify progression or recurrence, regular imaging investigations, blood tests, and skin exams are performed.

- **Management of Late Effects**: keeping an eye out for treatment-related side effects such as organ damage and recurrent cancers.

- **Supportive Care**: Dealing with problems related to quality of life, such as managing side effects of treatment and providing psychological support.

Monitoring and Surveillance Techniques

Strategies for surveillance that work well include:

Clinical Evaluations: To track skin lesions, dermatologists perform routine evaluations.

Imaging: To identify extracutaneous involvement, periodic imaging investigations (CT, PET) should be performed.

Laboratory Tests: Blood tests to track hematologic parameters and find cancerous cells in circulation.

- **Patient Self-Examinations**: Teaching patients to examine themselves regularly and to report any lesions that appear or change.

Patient Instruction on the Course of the Illness

Patient education is essential for efficient care:

- **Understanding the Disease**: Patients need to be aware of the symptoms, chronic nature, and significance of therapy and follow-up adherence for mycosis fungoides.

- **Symptom Recognition**: Teaching patients how to identify signs of a developing illness or its repercussions.

Lifestyle Modifications: Advice on how to take care of your skin, stay away from triggers, and stay healthy in general to help your therapy work.

The significance of thorough and customized care of mycosis fungoides is emphasized in Chapter 5:

- **Staging and Classification**: Precise staging and treatment planning depend on the TNMB system.

A crucial tool for identifying lymph node involvement is the **Sentinel Lymph Node Biopsy**.

Prognostic Factors: Several variables affect prognosis and treatment choices, such as age, sex, race, and genetic markers.

Surveillance and Follow-up: To manage long-term outcomes and discover progression early, patient education and routine monitoring are crucial.

- **Personalised Medicine**: More individualized and successful treatments are being made possible by the combination of genetic screening and biomarkers.

This all-encompassing strategy guarantees that patients receive the best care possible, customized to meet their unique needs and the unique features of their disease.

CHAPTER 6

STRATEGIES FOR TREATMENT

Topical Treatments

Corticosteroids

The first-line treatment for early-stage mycosis fungoides is frequently topical corticosteroids. By lowering the immunological response in the afflicted areas, they aid in the reduction of inflammation and skin lesions. From mild to superpotent, there are many potency levels available, enabling customized treatment based on the location and severity of the lesions. Prolonged use may result in striae, telangiectasias, and thinning of the skin, among other negative effects. To reduce side effects, patients need to be informed about correct application methods and how crucial it is to follow prescription dosage guidelines.

Retinoids

Topical retinoids, which regulate cell proliferation and differentiation, are synthetic derivatives of vitamin A. One example of this is bexarotene. They work well to treat early-stage mycosis fungoides because they minimize lesion size and encourage the return of normal skin cell growth. Skin dryness, photosensitivity, and inflammation are typical adverse effects. Patients must wear sunscreen and limit their exposure to the sun while receiving therapy. It's essential to see a dermatologist regularly to assess reaction and modify the treatment plan as necessary.

Photomedicine

PUVA (UVA with Psoralen)

In PUVA, psoralen, a photosensitizing drug, is administered, and then UVA light exposure occurs. Since it causes malignant T-cells to undergo apoptosis, this therapy works well for mycosis fungoides cases including a large amount of skin involvement. Usually, two or three sessions of treatment are held each week. Long-term use may result in side effects such as nausea, itching, and an elevated risk of skin cancer. After ingesting psoralen, patients must wear UVA-protective eyewear to shield their eyes from light exposure.

UVB

Another treatment option for mycosis fungoides in its early stages is broadband UVB phototherapy. It doesn't need a photosensitizing agent and is less intense than PUVA. UVB contributes to the inhibition of aberrant T-cell proliferation in the skin. Treatment is administered on a similar schedule to PUVA, with multiple treatment sessions each week. Reactions resembling sunburn as well as a long-term risk of skin ageing and cancer are possible adverse effects.

Narrow-Band UVB

When compared to broadband UVB, narrow-band UVB (NB-UVB) uses a particular wavelength of

UVB light (311-313 nm) that is more effective and has fewer adverse effects. For early-stage mycosis fungoides, NB-UVB is frequently recommended because of its tailored effect and decreased burning risk. Frequent treatments are required, and precautions against overexposure to UV radiation should be taken.

Systemic Interventions

Retinoids

When topical therapies are insufficient or for more severe stages of mycosis fungoides, systemic retinoids, like bexarotene, are utilized. They function by influencing gene expression and encouraging cancerous cells to undergo apoptosis. Liver dysfunction, hypothyroidism, and hyperlipidemia are possible side effects. Throughout treatment, it is crucial to regularly check thyroid function and blood lipid levels.

Methotrexine

Methotrexate is an immunosuppressive medication that prevents DNA synthesis, which stops cancerous T-cells from proliferating. Patients with more advanced or resistant mycosis fungoides are usually the ones who utilize it. Liver toxicity, bone marrow suppression, and gastrointestinal problems are possible side effects. To identify any negative effects early, patients need to be closely monitored and have regular blood tests.

Agents Biologics

Interferons

Cytokines called interferons, such as interferon-alpha, improve the immune system's defense against cancerous cells. They can be used either alone or in conjunction with other therapies to treat resistant or advanced mycosis fungoides. Hematologic abnormalities, tiredness, and flu-like symptoms are common adverse effects. It takes routine follow-up to control adverse effects and modify dosages.

Antibodies Monoclonal

Monoclonal antibodies that specifically target and destroy cancer T-cell antigens include mogamulizumab and alemtuzumab. These medications are used to treat Sézary syndrome or mycosis fungoides in advanced stages. Infections, cytopenias, and infusion responses are examples of side effects. Evaluation before therapy and continuous observation are essential for reducing risks and guaranteeing patient safety.

Radiation Treatment

Radiation from External Beams

By applying high-energy X-rays to the afflicted skin areas, external beam radiation treatment (EBRT) successfully lowers the tumor load. It is applied to localized lesions or, in more advanced stages, as a palliative measure to relieve symptoms. Fatigue, ulceration, and skin erythema are possible side effects. Precise targeting is part of treatment planning to reduce harm to nearby healthy tissues.

TSEBT, or total skin electron beam therapy

TSEBT involves treating the entire skin surface with electron beams. It can significantly control the disease and is quite effective for large skin involvement. Dryness of the skin, erythema, and transient hair loss are among the side effects. Additionally, patients may need supportive care both during and after therapy due to exhaustion. To monitor any long-term effects and evaluate response, regular follow-up is crucial.

Considerations for Stem Cell Transplantation

Patients with severe or refractory mycosis fungoides who have not responded to alternative therapy may be candidates for stem cell transplantation (SCT). Autologous and allogeneic transplants are available, with the possibility of a graft-versus-tumor impact with allogeneic stem cell transplantation. Eligibility requirements, illness condition, and organ function are all evaluated before transplantation. Managing problems like graft-versus-host disease (GVHD), infections, and relapse monitoring are all part of post-transplant care. Durable remission can be achieved with SCT, but long-term monitoring and careful patient selection are necessary.

Symptomatic Management and Supportive Care

Patients with mycosis fungoides need supportive treatment to improve their quality of life and manage their symptoms. This covers treating pruritus, taking care of the skin, and managing discomfort. Analgesics, emollients, and antihistamines are frequently utilized. Patients can manage the emotional and psychological effects of the illness with the assistance of psychological care and counseling. Comprehensive management greatly benefits from the involvement of multidisciplinary care teams, which include dermatologists, oncologists, and palliative care specialists.

Alternative Methods and Integrative Medicine

Acupuncture, mindfulness, and dietary changes are examples of integrative medicine techniques that may offer more symptom relief and enhance general health. Conventional treatments should be supplemented by these procedures, not substituted. Before implementing alternative therapies, patients should speak with their healthcare providers to be sure they won't conflict with prescribed medications. Integrative, evidence-based methods can improve patients' overall care.

Experimental Therapies and Clinical Trials

Access to novel and cutting-edge mycosis fungoides treatments is made possible by clinical trials. Patients can receive state-of-the-art treatments and support medical research by taking part in clinical trials. Novel biologics, targeted medicines, and combination regimens are examples of investigational treatments. Patients should think about the requirements for participation in a trial and explore the possible advantages and hazards with their healthcare practitioners. For therapy choices to advance and patient outcomes to improve, research must carry on.

An in-depth review of mycosis fungoides treatment approaches is given in Chapter 6, emphasizing the value of personalized, interdisciplinary care. Every technique, from radiation therapy to supportive care, and from topical therapies to systemic treatments, has its advantages and disadvantages. Clinical studies and newly developed therapies are broadening the therapeutic horizon and providing hope for better results. Improving patient care and quality of life requires a comprehensive strategy that incorporates supportive, conventional, and experimental therapy.

CHAPTER 7

HANDLING OF DIFFICULTIES

A form of cutaneous T-cell lymphoma known as mycosis fungoides (MF) is distinguished by the skin's accumulation of malignant T-cells. Improving patient outcomes and quality of life depends critically on the management of complications resulting from MF and its treatments. An in-depth summary of the important elements of MF complication management is given in this handbook.

Cutaneous Adverse Reactions to Medication

Synopsis

Because topical medications, phototherapy, and systemic medicines are used in MF treatments, cutaneous adverse events (CAEs) are frequently experienced. These can vary from minor skin irritation to serious reactions that impair the quality of life and adherence of the patient.

Frequent Adverse Occurrences

1. **Skin irritation and dermatitis**: Usually brought on by retinoids and topical steroids.

2. **Photosensitivity**: A side effect of phototherapy, such as PUVA.

3. **Infections**: More vulnerable to fungal, viral, and bacterial infections.

4. **Hyperpigmentation and Hypopigmentation**: Skin color changes brought on by extended therapy.

Techniques of Management

- **Prevention and Monitoring**: Conduct routine skin examinations to look for early indications of CAEs.

- **Symptomatic Treatment**: To control symptoms, use antihistamines, corticosteroids, and emollients.

Modifications to the Treatment: Changing therapy or adjusting dosages to lessen side effects.

- **Patient Education**: Educating patients on self-care techniques and any adverse effects.

Infections in Patients with Fungoides Mycosis

Synopsis

Because of their immunosuppressive therapies and poor skin barriers, patients with MF are more susceptible to infections.

Infection Types

- **Bacterial Infections**: Impetigo and cellulitis are frequent.

- **Viral Infections**: Zoster and herpes simplex.

- **Fungal Infections**: Dermatophyte infections and candidiasis.

Preventive and Administrative

- **Antimicrobial Prophylaxis**: Treating high-risk patients with prophylactic antibiotics, antivirals, or antifungals.

- **Hygiene Practices**: Stressing the need to take care of the skin and treating small wounds and abrasions right away.

Vaccinations: Maintaining current immunizations, especially for viral illnesses.

Early Detection and Treatment: Infections should be identified and treated as soon as possible to avoid consequences.

Hematologic Problems (Leukopenia, Anaemia)

Synopsis

Hematologic problems can develop as a side effect of chemotherapy or as a result of the disease itself.

Kinds of Difficulties

Anaemia: A low red blood cell count that causes weakness and exhaustion.

Leukopenia: Reduced white blood cell count raising the possibility of infection.

Techniques of Management

- **Regular Monitoring**: Regular blood work to identify hematologic abnormalities in advance.

- **Supportive Treatments**: Iron supplements, blood transfusions, and the use of growth factors.

Treatment Adjustments: Making changes to or halting prescription regimens that increase the risk of hematotoxicity.

Needs for Emotional and Psychological Support

Synopsis

Patients may require psychological and emotional support because of the chronic nature of MF and its therapies, which can have a substantial negative influence on their mental health.

Typical Problems

Depression and Anxiety: As a result of the disease's recurrent and chronic character.

- **Body Image Concerns**: Caused by scars and noticeable skin blemishes.

Handling the psychological impact of a long-term medical condition: **Stress and Coping Challenges**.

Strategies of Support

Frequent meetings with a psychologist or psychiatrist constitute **Psychological Counselling**.

- **Support Groups**: Making connections with those going through comparable struggles.

Mind-Body Techniques: Mindfulness, yoga, and meditation are examples of such practices.

- **Family Support**: Including family members as a support network throughout the caregiving process.

Nutritional Factors to Take Into Account

Synopsis

For MF patients, maintaining overall health and controlling treatment adverse effects depend on proper nutrition.

Dietary Difficulties

- **Malnutrition**: As a result of therapeutic side effects or a diminished appetite.

- **Specific Nutrient Deficiencies**: Anaemia caused by an iron deficit, for example.

Dietary Techniques

- **Dietary Assessment**: A dietician will regularly assess you.

- **Balanced Diet**: To promote energy levels and immunological function, a nutrient-rich diet is stressed.

Supplements: Remedial of specific deficits through the use of vitamins and minerals.

Hydration: Make sure you're getting enough fluids in.

Techniques for Pain Management

Synopsis

Because of the skin lesions, treatments, and other problems associated with MF, pain management is essential.

Pain Causes

- **Skin Lesions**: Sore spots and ulcers that hurt.

- **Side Effects of Treatment**: Radiation or chemotherapy pain.

Methods of Pain Management

- **Topical Analgesics**: Ointments and creams for the localization of pain.

NSAIDs, paracetamol, and opioids for more severe pain are **Systemic Analgesics**.

- **Non-Pharmacological Methods**: Methods like physical therapy, cognitive-behavioral therapy, and acupuncture.

- **Multidisciplinary Approach**: Including dermatologists, pain management specialists, and primary care physicians.

Risk of Second Malignancy and Monitoring

Synopsis

Patients with MF are more likely to experience immunosuppression and mutagenic therapies, which can lead to recurrent cancers.

Frequent Secondary Cancers

Other types of lymphoma, or **Non-Hodgkin Lymphoma**.

Cancers of the skin: Squamous cell carcinoma and Basal cell carcinoma.

- **Solid Tumours**: These comprise malignancies of the breast, colon, and lungs.

Monitoring Techniques

- **Regular Screenings**: laboratory testing, imaging studies, and dermatologic examinations.

- **Risk Factor Modification**: Dealing with changeable risk factors like quitting smoking and wearing sunscreen.

Patient Education: Educating patients on the warning signs and symptoms of cancers that come back later in life.

Handling Problems with Life Quality

Synopsis

Considering that MF is a chronic condition, improving quality of life (QoL) is a top priority in its management.

Important QoL Concerns

- **Physical Symptoms**: Handling weariness, soreness, and itching.

Psychological Impact: Dealing with concerns related to mental health.

- **Social and Occupational Challenges**: Handling the effects on day-to-day activities and employment.

Methods to Boost Quality of Life

- **Comprehensive Symptom Management**: Efficiently handling bodily symptoms.

- **Psychological Services**: Availability for mental health support.

- **Social Support Services**: Help with professional and social obstacles.

Patient-Centered Care: Making decisions with patients to match treatments to their preferences and way of life.

Talks on Palliative Care and End-of-Life Issues

Synopsis

Palliative treatment is aimed at relieving MF symptoms and associated stress, particularly when the disease is advanced.

Elements of Palliative Care

-    **Symptom   Management**:   Managing discomforting symptoms such as pain and nausea.

Offering spiritual and emotional support is known as **Psychosocial Support**.

- **Advance Care Planning**: Talking about and recording patients' preferences for care towards the end of life.

- **Interdisciplinary Approach**: Using a group of medical professionals to handle different demands.

Conversations Regarding Dying

- **Honest Communication**: Giving caring, understandable facts regarding the prognosis and available treatments.

- **Family Support**: Helping families comprehend and manage end-of-life concerns.

- **Hospice Care**: Whenever necessary, transferring to hospice care to guarantee comfort and dignity.

Recap of Managing Complications

Synopsis

To effectively manage problems in MF, a multidisciplinary strategy that takes into account the social, psychological, and physical aspects of care is required.

Important Details

Early Detection and Intervention: Consistent observation and timely intervention in case of difficulties.

- **Multidisciplinary Care**: Coordinating efforts between medical professionals to treat difficult cases.

Patient Education and Involvement: Giving patients information and allowing them to participate in choosing their medical care.

- **Supportive and Palliative Care**: Providing emotional support and symptom management to maintain quality of life.

Healthcare professionals may greatly improve patient outcomes and the general quality of life for people with MF by taking a proactive and holistic approach to managing complications in the condition. MF is a chronic and difficult disorder.

CHAPTER 8

VIEWS FROM PATIENTS AND CARERS

Advocacy and Empowerment of Patients

Comprehending the PrognosisSkin T-cell lymphoma in the rare form of Mycosis Fungoides (MF). Understanding the nature of MF, its stages, and available treatments is essential because "knowledge is power." Look for reliable sources and educate yourself so that you may choose wisely.

Promotion and Self-Promotion

Being an advocate means taking an active role in your treatment. Participate in awareness campaigns, join patient advocacy groups, and work with MF-focused organizations. Being a self-advocate entails speaking with confidence to your healthcare team about your needs and preferences.

Resources and Rights:

Learn about your rights as a patient, which include the ability to view your medical information, the ability to get a second opinion, and the right to be treated with dignity and respect. Use patient advocacy groups and other resources as a source of information and support.

Patient Coping Techniques

Psychological Health:

Finding out you have MF can be very upsetting. Feeling a variety of emotions is normal, such as fear, rage, and sadness. To better handle these emotions, think about obtaining treatment or counseling.

Handling Stress

Engage in stress-reduction practices including yoga, deep breathing exercises, meditation, and mindfulness. These can lessen anxiety and enhance general well-being.

Aiding Organisations

Getting involved in support groups helps foster a feeling of belonging and mutual understanding. Making connections with people who have gone through similar things can provide both practical guidance and emotional support.

Lifestyle Adjustments for Improved Health

Nutrition and Diet

Keep a diet full of whole grains, fruits, veggies, lean meats, and other nutrients. Some meals can strengthen your immune system and enhance your general health. Seek advice from a nutritionist to create a customized eating schedule.

Activity Outside

Frequent exercise improves both mental and physical health. Whenever possible, try to get in at least 30 minutes of moderate exercise most days of the week, unless your doctor instructs you otherwise.

Healthy Routines

Refrain from smoking and drink in moderation. Maintaining a regular sleep schedule and setting up a peaceful sleeping environment are examples of good sleep hygiene.

Interacting with Medical Professionals

Skillful Interaction:

Communicate honestly and openly with your medical team. Ask questions when you have them prepared, and don't be afraid to clarify anything you don't understand.

Establishing a ConnectionEstablish a rapport based on trust with your medical professionals. Inform them regularly about your symptoms, side effects, and any modifications to your health.

Awareness:

Keep yourself updated about recent advancements in MF research as well as your treatment options. This makes it possible for you to have insightful conversations with your medical staff.

Actively Using Support Systems

Friends and Family:

Rely on loved ones and friends for both practical and emotional help. Inform them about your condition and the course of your treatment.

Resources for Community:

Investigate online and local support systems, such as social services, community health organizations, and patient advocacy groups.

Colleague Assistance:

Use internet forums or support organizations to establish connections with other MF patients. It can be quite beneficial to exchange experiences and suggestions.

Resources for Support and Difficulties for Carers

Understanding the Roles of Carers:

To provide both physical and emotional support, carers are essential. Recognize the obligations and challenges that come with providing care.

Carers' Self-Care:

In addition, carers need to put their health and wellbeing first. Take pauses, look for temporary help, and think about joining support groups for carers.

Carers' Resources:

Make use of resources like financial aid, counseling services, and carer education programs. Several resources are available for carers through organizations like the American Cancer Society.

Making Decisions with the Patient in Mind

Educated Decisions:

Make choices after carefully considering your diagnosis, available treatments, and possible results. Examine a variety of sources and, if needed, seek second viewpoints.

Signature Ideals:

When making decisions, keep your values, preferences, and objectives in mind. Make sure that your priorities and way of life are reflected in your treatment plan.

Involved Engagement:

Take an active role in all aspects of your care, including controlling side effects and choosing your course of treatment. This encourages empowerment and a sense of control.

Collaborative Decision-Making in Therapy Plans

Cooperative Method:

In shared decision-making, you and your healthcare team work together. Reach a decision that honors your choices after discussing the advantages and disadvantages of each of your treatment alternatives.

Resources and Tools:

To better grasp your alternatives, make use of decision aids including brochures, websites, and videos. These resources can help you and your healthcare providers have more fruitful conversations.

Ongoing Evaluation:

Review your treatment plan regularly with your medical team. Be willing to make changes in response to new information, shifting conditions, or shifting desires.

Motivational Tales and Testimonials from Patients

Actual Life Encounters:

Gaining insight from those who have experienced comparable journeys can be immensely inspiring. Testimonials and anecdotes that inspire hope emphasize perseverance and provide useful insights.

Acquired Knowledge:

Learn from other people's experiences, including the difficulties they had and the solutions they found. This can offer insightful perspective and motivation.

Link with the Community:

Talking with other patients about their experiences helps to create a feeling of shared experience and community. It serves as a reminder that you are not traveling alone.

CHAPTER 9

PROSPECTIVE ROUTES AND ONCOMING TREATMENTS

Developments in Immunotherapy

Immunotherapy has transformed the way that many malignancies, including mycosis fungoides (MF), are treated. The goal of recent developments is to use the immune system of the body to identify and eliminate cancer cells. Checkpoint inhibitors, such as CTLA-4 and PD-1 blockers, have demonstrated potential in boosting the body's defenses against myeloid-derived macrophages. These treatments aid in defeating the immune evasion strategies that cancer cells use. Furthermore, research is being done on adoptive cell therapies, such as CAR-T cell therapy. These entail modifying the T-cells of patients to more effectively identify and combat cancer cells, potentially providing individualized and very successful therapy choices.

Precision Medicine and Targeted Therapies

The goal of targeted therapy is to precisely block the molecular mechanisms that fuel the growth and survival of cancer. Treatments for MF are being developed that specifically target abnormal signaling pathways and certain mutations. For instance, clinical trials have demonstrated the effectiveness of inhibitors of the JAK/STAT pathway, which is frequently dysregulated in MF. Treatment plans in precision medicine are customized according to the genetic and molecular characteristics of each patient's tumor. By choosing the medicines that are most likely to be helpful for each patient based on their specific tumor features, this strategy offers less harmful and more effective treatments.

Applications of Nanotechnology in Dermatology

Novel techniques for the diagnosis and treatment of MF are provided by nanotechnology. Drugs can be delivered to cancer cells directly using nanoparticle engineering, reducing systemic side effects and increasing treatment efficacy. Therapeutic drugs can be delivered precisely with these nanoparticles since they can be engineered to target specific molecules expressed in MF cells. Furthermore, nanotechnology can enhance imaging methods, enabling earlier diagnosis and better tracking of the course of a disease. Research is being done to create theranostic nanoparticles, which combine therapeutic and diagnostic properties, and nanocarriers for different anti-cancer medications.

Artificial Intelligence for the Handling of Diseases

With its ability to improve diagnostic precision, forecast treatment results, and customize patient care, artificial intelligence (AI) is revolutionizing disease management in MF. Large datasets containing clinical, histological, and genomic data can be analyzed using machine learning algorithms to find trends and biomarkers linked to the course of a disease and its response to treatment. By enhancing the interpretation of skin biopsies and imaging investigations, artificial intelligence can help with early diagnosis. Additionally, by offering suggestions based on real-time data analysis and predictive modeling, AI-driven solutions can assist clinical decision-making and eventually improve patient outcomes.

Innovations in Regenerative Medicine

Patients with MF may benefit from regenerative medicine's potential to repair damaged skin and enhance their quality of life. The goal of methods like tissue engineering and stem cell treatment is to rebuild healthy skin tissue. Mesenchymal stem cells (MSCs) can be employed to stimulate tissue healing and reduce inflammation because of their immunomodulatory qualities. Furthermore, improvements in bioengineering are making it possible to create scaffolds and skin grafts that can be used to replace damaged skin. Although these developments are still in the experimental phase, they provide hope for longer-lasting and more efficient treatments for MF-related skin damage.

Research on Patient-Reported Outcomes

Awareness of the effects of MF and its therapies on patients' quality of life requires an awareness of patient-reported outcomes or PROs. Direct patient data collection regarding symptoms, treatment outcomes, and general well-being is a key component of PRO research. With the use of this information, medical professionals can better customize patient care to meet their unique requirements and preferences in addition to the disease. PROs are being added to clinical studies more frequently to make sure that novel treatments help patients. This method places a strong emphasis on patient-centered care and may result in more all-encompassing and successful treatment plans.

Initiatives for Health Equity and Access to Care

Ensuring access to care and health fairness is essential to improve MF outcomes. For some patient populations, disparities in access to modern treatments, diagnostic equipment, and healthcare services can result in less favorable outcomes. Expanding healthcare coverage, boosting funding for community health programs, and encouraging consumer and healthcare provider education and awareness regarding MF are among the initiatives being taken to address these inequities. In addition, telemedicine and mobile health technologies can help reach underprivileged groups and give them prompt access to specialized care and specialists.

International Partnerships for Research on Mycosis Fungoides

Research on MF must be advanced internationally to create novel treatments. Researchers can speed up the development of new medicines and deepen their understanding of disease mechanisms by exchanging data, resources, and expertise. Global research networks and multinational clinical trials are two examples of collaborative efforts that make it easier to acquire a variety of patient data, which can produce conclusions that are more broadly applicable. International collaborations can also aid in standardizing treatment protocols and enhancing global access to state-of-the-art treatments.

Schedule of Upcoming Clinical Trials

To progress in the field, MF should prioritize many important topics for future clinical trials. Among them are:

1. **Combination Therapies**: Research how well various treatment methods, including

immunotherapy, targeted therapy, and conventional treatments, can be combined to improve therapeutic results.

2. **Biomarker Development**: To enable more individualized treatment methods, biomarkers for predicting therapy response and illness progression must be found and validated.

3. **Long-term Outcomes**: Carrying out long-term research to evaluate the influence on overall survival and quality of life, as well as the durability of treatment responses.

4. **Paediatric and Geriatric Populations**: Ensuring that medicines are safe and effective for all patients by including a range of age groups in clinical trials.

5. **Real-world Evidence**: Combining information from actual clinical settings to support results from controlled clinical trials and shed light on how well therapies work in everyday healthcare environments.

Prospects for Mycosis Fungoides

There are a lot of exciting developments in MF research and therapy in the works. More efficient and individualized treatment options are anticipated as long as immunotherapy, targeted treatments, and precision medicine continue to innovate. AI and other emerging technologies will improve illness management and diagnostic capacities. Novel treatments will be tailored to the various needs of patients through cooperative research endeavors and a patient-centered care emphasis. The field may strive to guarantee that all patients benefit from these developments by placing a high priority on health equity and access to care, which will eventually improve outcomes and quality of life for people with MF.

CHAPTER 10

SUMMARY OF CRUCIAL INFORMATION

A kind of cutaneous T-cell lymphoma known as mycosis fungoides (MF) has an indolent history but has the potential to advance to more severe stages. Understanding its clinical appearance, which frequently starts with patch and plaque stages before possibly progressing to tumors and systemic involvement, is one of the key pieces of information. Complex diagnosis frequently necessitates blood testing, imaging scans, and skin biopsies. Depending on the disease's stage and severity, treatment options range from skin-directed therapies (such as topical steroids, and phototherapy) to systemic treatments (such as chemotherapy, and biologics).

Value of Multidisciplinary Medical Care

A multidisciplinary strategy combining dermatologists, oncologists, pathologists, radiologists, and occasionally additional specialists like hematologists and radiation oncologists is necessary for the effective care of MF. This cooperative endeavor guarantees all-encompassing treatment, attending to both the illness and the patient's general state of health. It supports the precise diagnosis, customized therapy planning, and ongoing observation for possible side effects or consequences from treatment.

Empowerment and Education of Patients

It is essential to arm people with information regarding their disease. Patients need to be informed about the causes of muscle fibrosis (MF), available treatments, possible adverse effects, and the value of routine follow-up visits. Giving patients access to tools like factual brochures, support groups, and trustworthy websites can help them make better decisions about their care and enhance their quality of life.

Needs for Further Research

To better understand the pathophysiology of MF, enhance diagnostic methods, and create more potent medications with fewer adverse effects, additional research is necessary. The molecular and genetic components of MF are the focus of current research, which may result in tailored treatment plans and targeted medications. It is important to promote clinical trial participation to further these developments.

Supporting the Mycosis Fungoides Society

To increase patient care, research funding, and public knowledge of MF are all made possible in large part through advocacy. Encouraging groups that fight for patients with MF and taking part in advocacy campaigns can make a big difference in the community by bringing about improved services and support networks for individuals impacted.

Recognition and Expressions of Thanks

The committed medical experts, researchers, and support personnel who contribute to the treatment and expansion of MF knowledge should all be acknowledged. Patients and their families who take part in clinical trials and research, paving the way for future improvements, too deserve gratitude.

Referrals and Evaluations

The reliability and usefulness of the guide are confirmed by the positive recommendations of healthcare organizations, patient testimonies, and professional endorsements. These testimonials highlight the guide's worth as a reliable resource for medical professionals and patients alike.

How to Keep Up with Developments in Mycosis Fungoides

Keeping up with the most recent advancements in MF can be accomplished by subscribing to medical journals, becoming a member of professional societies, and attending dermatology and oncology-focused conferences and webinars. Reputable organizations' newsletters and online platforms offer frequent information on new research discoveries, therapy recommendations, and clinical trial chances.

Closing Remarks and Motivation

Although managing MF might be difficult, there is promise for improved outcomes and management thanks to medical science developments. Patients are urged to take an active role in their care, communicate openly with their medical staff, and look to their loved ones and community for support. For those suffering from MF, there appears to be hope for the future with ongoing research and teamwork in care.

Glossary of Terms
Appendix

- **Cutaneous T-cell lymphoma (CTCL):** A non-Hodgkin lymphoma, originating from the skin's T-cells.

Indolent: slowly spreading or posing minimal discomfort.

- **Biopsy:** A diagnostic procedure in which tissues or cells are extracted for analysis.

- **Phototherapy:** Light therapy, frequently employed to address skin ailments.

- **Biologics:** Drugs used to treat a range of illnesses that are derived from living things.

Pathogenesis: The beginning and progression of an illness.

Clinical trial: Experiments conducted on humans to assess behavioral, surgical, or medicinal therapies.

By offering thorough knowledge and assistance to individuals impacted by mycosis fungoides, this guide hopes to promote a better comprehension and more efficient treatment of the illness.